Introduction

We love capsule wardrobes.

We love creating them and we love the ease of getting dressed when everything in our wardrobe works well together and works well for our lifestyle.

We love shopping our wardrobes to see what we have at the beginning of each season and we love creating a truly functional wardrobe from what we have, before we hit the shops.

But, before capsule wardrobes became 'a thing' we were both like many people out there; a wardrobe bursting at the seams with 'nothing to wear' and shopping for the perfect item that was not quite that perfect when we got it home.

Sound familiar?

Do you have a wardrobe jam packed with clothes? Do you stand in front of your wardrobe every morning and announce you have nothing to wear?

Do you look at all those girls on YouTube, Instagram and blogs who show you how to put together the perfect wardrobe - after you've spent a fortune on designer pieces?

Do you own some of the pieces they recommend, but when you put them on you don't feel great? You pull and tug and just feel generally uncomfortable?

That was us!

And then we realised we weren't like those young and gorgeous Instagrammers. We were real women; with families, budgets and no gifts from designers being couriered to our door.

So, we have created this guide to share with you; a way for a real woman, with a real life and a real budget to create a capsule wardrobe that works for her.

Chapter 1

Analysing Your Style

Before you can plan your perfect, or perfect for you, capsule wardrobe, you first must work out who you really are. This chapter is about making sure YOUR style is acknowledged and that YOUR capsule wardrobe reflects the individual you.

Having the right clothes in your wardrobe will make all the difference to loving what you wear each day, so ask yourself these questions;

- How do I spend my days?
- Do my clothes suit my life right now?
- What do I wear, and what should I be wearing, every day?
- Do I have an identifiable uniform?

Let's look at the answers to these questions and how they help to create a capsule wardrobe that is just right for you.

How Do You Spend Your Days?

Are you a part time or fulltime at home mum or are you a fulltime working woman? Are you a college/university student or have you retired?

A fulltime working woman has different wardrobe needs than a part time working mum and different again to a full-time student or a retired lady with grown children. Each woman needs a wardrobe that functions for her lifestyle; her day to day life, working life, social commitments and family commitments.

You will need to give some thought to the different ways you spend your day and the different types of clothes you will need during the day.

Do Your Clothes Suit Your Life Right Now?

The fantasy you versus the real you: this is one of the easiest wardrobe mistakes to make and a trap that many of us have fallen into. It can sometimes be hard to identify or accept our real-life situation and say goodbye to the clothes that dress our fantasy self or the person we used to be.

We sometimes buy clothes to dress the person we want to be, not the person we are now;

- Being a student but buying clothes for our future career
- Buying dresses for a social life that doesn't eventuate
- Buying stilettos when our lifestyle favours lower heels
- Wearing skirts because, well, doesn't everyone, shouldn't we?
- Buying a little black dress or a crisp white blouse because all the style books say we must.

It's good to have life and career goals and aspirations but buying and keeping clothes now for a fantasy or future you, doesn't help you get dressed every morning in your current life.

Ellen says: My fantasy self meets my husband in the city after work for drinks at a swanky bar. The real me is a mum of two school age children, who runs a small business from home. Cocktail dresses are not a reality right now, so I focus my energy (and budget!) on cute outfits that suit my life exactly as it is today.

Claire says: My fantasy self works in a more corporate environment than I really do. I work in an office part time and need smart casual clothes and practical shoes with a medium heel. My fantasy self loves designer tailored suits and shoes with killer heels and pointed toes.

What Do You Wear Every Day?

What is your go to outfit?
 What types of clothes make you feel good?
Which of your outfits get the most compliments?

Do you prefer;

- jeans and boots?
- skirts and flats?
- long skirts or short skirts?
- pants all the time?
- jeans and a flannel shirt?
- ruffles, frills and heels?

Are the clothes that you are choosing to wear practical, suitable, comfortable and realistic or do you struggle daily to get your job done, hampered by unsuitable outfits?

What Should You Be Wearing?

For example; heels and tailored suits make life in a child care centre hard, jeans and a casual blouse are not usually suitable attire for a corporate environment and at the end of the day, many of us won't feel comfortable.

While these are obvious and exaggerated examples, identifying the clothes you need to wear and how many days of the week you need these clothes is one of the first steps in identifying the needs of your ideal capsule wardrobe.

Do You Wear A Uniform?

Do you reach for the same style of clothes every day?

Being able to see a pattern in your clothing choices when you look in the wardrobe, or think about what you've worn recently, is going to make creating a capsule wardrobe that much easier.

Your 'uniform' is the outfit that;

- you wear daily because it makes you feel comfortable
- is acceptable in your daily environment
- expresses your personality
- makes you feel like 'you'

Claire says: Once I had children I gave up wearing skirts. They just weren't practical and didn't suit my post baby figure. Now I almost always wear pants. To work I wear tailored pants and a form fitting three quarter sleeve top. I've found that having broad shoulders and a high waist, button down shirts just don't work for me. A knit style top fits nicely across the shoulders and is comfortable for computer work. My preference is then to top that with a cardigan, most often in the same colour as the pants, giving me a softly structured suit like appearance. Low heeled loafers or a medium heel dress shoe finishes my 'uniform'.

Ellen says: My personal 'uniform' is jeans with a top and a topper. I wear jeans in several different shades and cuts to give my look variety. My tops are usually plain or striped and the toppers I love are padded vests and long-line cardigans. I don't wear much jewellery, so I often like to wear a scarf to add interest to my outfit.

What If I Can't Identify My Uniform?

If you can't identify a uniform just yet, don't worry. Consider the following words; can you find two or three words, or maybe others not on the list, that reflect how you would describe yourself and then see if they are reflected in your wardrobe.

romantic	casual	resort
Floral	professional	corporate
formal	down to earth	tailored
soft	rockabilly	modest
flowing	trendy	sleek
hippy	comfortable	natural
straight	classic	modern
arty	hipster	sporty
boho	ethical	carefree
cute	streamlined	float
trendy	chic	French
nautical	country	retro
simple	pattern	modern
elegant	monochrome	minimalist
quirky	structured	

Still not sure what your uniform or style might be? After thinking about what you wear and looking at the descriptive words, look in your wardrobe again and consider the following.

- Think about your 'go to outfit', the one you reach for all the time.
- Look at some recent photos and take note of what you're wearing.
- Do you have favourite pieces you always reach for?
- If someone else was to describe you, what outfit would they put you in? Is this the 'real you' or are you reaching for anything, so you don't do school drop off in your pyjamas.
- In a shop, what silhouettes, colours and styles do you gravitate towards?

Ask your partner, work colleague, friend or a family member how they would describe the way you dress. Do they all come up with similar answers?

Another way to identify your style is to start a Pinterest board or scrapbook and pin or stick in any images that catch your eye. With so many outfit options available on line and in print media, what you first gravitate towards and what you avoid, can tell you a lot about your personal style.

Once you have as selection, assess them with a critical eye. Can you see similarities in the images you have selected?

Chapter 1 Summary

Do you wear the right clothes for the way you spend your day?

Are there too many clothes in your wardrobe that dress the fantasy you?

When you look at your clothes, can you see a 'uniform'?

Chapter 1 Activities

The sorts of clothes I need to wear daily include;

_____

_____

Words that describe my style include;

_____

_____

I'd describe my uniform as;

_____

_____

_____

Chapter 2

Behind Closed Doors

What's in your wardrobe?
Now it's time to have a closer look at what's behind those wardrobe doors. Before you put together your ideal capsule wardrobe, you might need to do a little decluttering and get rid of some items that really shouldn't be in your wardrobe.

When you open your wardrobe, what do you see? A jumble, a rainbow of colours, basic black, empty coat hangers or military precision? Do the items in there reflect the current you and the style or uniform you have identified?

Are there items in there from a past life or your fantasy life?

- clothes that you wore pre-kids
- at school or college
- the graduation ball
- fat clothes
- thin clothes
- maternity clothes

- fantasy you
- bridesmaid's dresses
- unworn clothes
- and things you wished you had never bought?

Let's Get To It

On a free day, (because this will take longer than you think), take everything out of your wardrobe until it is totally empty. Pile everything onto the bed or the floor and take a long hard look at it all. As you sort through your clothes, separate summer and winter items.

Pack away the clothes that aren't relevant. Knowing what it is going to be like outside for the next season and if you can, pack away the clothes you will not need into a suitcase, a storage tub or a spare room wardrobe.

This is an easy step. You don't need to make any decision about an item of clothing other than 'is this piece suitable for this season?' If it's winter, then swimwear can be put away or if it's summer, the woollen coat isn't needed. If you are heading into a transitional season you might not yet be able to decide which long or short sleeve tops and which shorts or pants you want to keep out.

If it isn't a clear YES or NO keep the clothes out as you continue to define and refine your needs.

Now it's time for three piles; yes, no, maybe.

Pick up each item and as you hold it in your hand decide;

Yes - I love it and wear it often

No - I don't like it, don't wear it, it doesn't fit, what was I thinking!

Maybe - but I'm not sure. I might if I had something to wear it with, the hem has come down, it needs a button moved etc.

Hang up the clothes from your yes pile, these will be the basis of your capsule wardrobe and we will get to them in a minute.
Bag up those you no longer like or wear and get them out of the house.

- donate them to a charity shop
- donate them to a women's refuge or shelter
- sell them via eBay, Gumtree, Facebook or a consignment store (see the reference section for a 'how to sell on line' guide)
- the bin or the ragbag, if they are truly unwearable

The Maybe Pile.

Now to the 'maybe' pile. This may take a bit longer to work through.

Select one item at a time and critically assess it and imagine how it fits into your life today.

How would you feel if you got rid of it and didn't see it again? Let there be no guilt in your wardrobe, learn from your mistakes and move forward.

Yes, you've spent money on items, but leaving them hanging unworn in your wardrobe won't make you feel any better about the purchase. In fact, every time you look at that item you feel the guilt all over again.

For many people, some items of clothing often have negative feelings attached to them and there is often a great sense of relief to get rid of those clothes.

Set aside those that you want to keep that need repairing. Get it done or take it to someone that can do it for you (Hi Mum!).

Those that you are not sure about box up and store them somewhere for six months. If you need an item, you know where it is and can go and get it.

If you've not needed anything in that time and have even forgotten what in the box, don't open it, drop it off at a charity shop next time you are going by.

Now that all the unloved and unworn clothes are no longer taking up space in your wardrobe, let's have a look at what's left;

- are you looking at your favourite clothes?
- are these the clothes you wear most of the time?
- does your uniform stand out? can you see your 'style' or even a hint of one?

- remember, it's quite okay if you don't have an identifiable style or uniform.

Seasonal Dressing

Another thing to consider, before you start selecting your own capsule wardrobe is the seasons where you live.

Creating a capsule wardrobe is not a definitive exercise and while there are plenty of people that live in temperate climates and can wear the same clothes all year, many of us tend to experience multiple seasons.

We will need to regularly change our wardrobes, by either having seasonal capsules that are totally different to the one before or gradually swapping items in and out as the seasons change.

Capsule wardrobes for autumn (fall) and spring can be referred to as *'transitional capsule wardrobes',* as they transition or move from one extreme (hot/cold) to the other (cold/hot). Additional planning for this wardrobe will be discussed in the next chapter.

Budget.

Finally, before we get into the fun part of creating our first capsule wardrobe, we need to talk about money. While this isn't a book about money it is important when updating or replacing your wardrobe that you don't have a budget blow out and overspend.

It is important and realistic to have a budget and to make the most of your purchases.

Set yourself a clothing budget; weekly, monthly or seasonally – make sure it aligns with your, and/or your family's, values and goals. Most of us don't have lavish lifestyles with limitless money (or brand sponsorship on Instagram!)

Often, when a family budget is considered, a mother puts her needs and wants last. If you are single or childfree, you may consider your investments, savings, travel or mortgage to be more important than personal purchases. But even a very small clothing budget gives you money you can spend on yourself without guilt and it helps you to maintain a well-dressed look.

A few dollars set aside each week or fortnight, either in a separate account or in a secret stash in your jewellery box, gives you the option to buy an item that you feel might be missing from your wardrobe.

Cost vs. Worth

This is a really important point to consider and to get your head around. The clothing in your wardrobe is worth a lot less than it cost you. This applies to most items in your home.

Just because you paid $100 for that black dress, once it is hanging in your wardrobe, worn or unworn, it is worth a lot less than that. No one will buy it from you for what you paid for it. It is now second hand, worn or not.

Perhaps you might consider everything in your wardrobe as being worth $0, then you don't have to feel any guilt or regret over past purchases, particularly if you plan to move them on.

The importance of cost versus worth is something to remember whenever you purchase anything.

Cost per Wear Ratio

Another important point to consider is the cost per wear ratio.

How often do we find something we love but put it back when we see the price?
Often we settle for something cheaper and then leave it hanging in the wardrobe, knowing it was our second choice.

A beautiful jacket that you love and that works well with your lifestyle and existing wardrobe might costs $200, but will turn out to cost less than the $10 top you found on the clearance rack that was a strange colour and pilled after its first wash that you stopped wearing.

A $200 jacket that lasts 10 years and is worn once a week every winter will cost $1.66 per wear;

 $200 divide by 10 years = $20 per year divided by 12 wears per winter (once a week) = $1.66 per wear

A $10 top that looked shabby after wearing and washing twice will cost $5 per wear;

$10 divide 2 wears = $5

While this is an extreme example, can you see that a more expensive item can be better value for money? As a bonus, every time you wear the jacket you will feel great and both times you wear the top you'll probably find yourself tugging and adjusting and generally feeling uncomfortable.

Chapter 2 Summary

Realistically assess your clothes dividing them into three groups; yes, no and maybe then pack away the clothes you won't be wearing this season.

Set a budget that is realistic for you and your situation. No matter how small, it's nice to have a little something set aside to update your wardrobe guilt free each season.

What an item cost you and what it is worth are not the same thing.

Cost per wear ration – even though an item might have been more expensive to purchase, the more you wear it, the better value for money it becomes.

Chapter 2 Activities

After sorting through my wardrobe and removing clothes that have made me feel guilty, I now feel;

_____

_____

_____

The best way for me to store my off season clothes is;

_____

_____

A realistic clothing budget for me is;

_____

_____

Are you able to work out the cost per wear ratio of an item of clothing you have worn regularly and compare it to the cost per wear ratio of something that probably wasn't such a good buy?

Chapter 3

Creating Your First Capsule Wardrobe

'Capsule wardrobe' is a term created by Susie Faux in the 1970's, the owner of 'Wardrobe' a London boutique.

She said that a capsule wardrobe is a collection of a few essential items of clothing that don't go out of fashion; such as skirts, trousers, and coats, which can then be added to with different pieces each season.

Your capsule wardrobe is a group of clothes that work well together to give optimum possibilities from the least number of items.

Now it's time to take what you've learnt earlier and put it into action.

If you consider all the key words and thoughts you have put together, can you look at them as a structure or framework to build a capsule wardrobe that suits you?

Your capsule wardrobe is not ten items a '20 something' blogger says you *must* own this season,

Nor is it a collection of designer clothes you cannot afford. (You don't think every fashion blogger buys all their own clothes, do you?)

It is important that you define *your own* capsule wardrobe that works for *your life,* and *your life* style.

Your location, budget, occupation and the local seasons play a major role in this wardrobe.

Transitional Capsule Wardrobes

The seasons where you live will greatly influence your capsule wardrobe. Some people may only need two capsules; one for warm weather and another for cool weather, but some will need four capsules to suit the varying climate where they live.

Seasons just don't start and end. Just because technically winter ended yesterday doesn't mean it is spring today. It is the third day of spring as we write this. It is grey and cloudy; it is trying to rain and only 16 degrees (59F), so we are still wearing clothes from our winter wardrobes.

Where we live, summer and winter are easily defined seasons and spring and autumn are more temperamental. These are called transition seasons as they lead from one extreme into another and in the transition seasons you will need to consider wider variations in temperature.

Here in southern Australia, we are coming out of winter, but it is not warm yet. We still need coats and boots, and then before we move into our summer capsule we will have moved from coats to long sleeves and then short sleeves. It is a gradual process as each wardrobe appears to evolve into the next.

Ellen says: Where I live there is a cold but not freezing winter (no snow), autumn and spring are both quite variable and can range from hot to cold and both usually have lots of rain. Summer here is hot, with a few weeks of very hot weather each year.

Claire says: I live further south than Ellen. We have similar seasonal patterns, but I have a slightly colder winter and milder summer. I have a small summer wardrobe and a much larger winter wardrobe that covers the variable spring and autumn days.

Core and Accent Colours

Now that your off-season clothes are packed away and the old, worn and unloved items have gone, it's time to talk about the next step in creating a capsule wardrobe – colour!

To make a cohesive wardrobe that works well, you need a selection of clothes that are complimentary. If it's not already obvious when you look in your wardrobe, then you need to decide on some colour combinations that work well for you and that you are happy to use as a base for creating your own capsule wardrobe.

Claire says: My core colour is navy blue. My neutral colour is cream, and my two accent colours are khaki and peach. These colours suit my colouring, work well together and were the dominant colours in my existing wardrobe. So, for me, the choice was easy. It doesn't mean I can't or won't wear any other colours, it means these are the ones I prefer to wear and am now building my wardrobe around them

Ellen says: I like more variety in my colour palette, but I still use the idea of core and accent colours to make sure my wardrobe pieces works well together. My core colours are black, denim and grey all year round. In each season I will add two or three accent colours which may repeat or change year to year. I spend more of my budget on more expensive core pieces and buy cheap fun trendy pieces as my accent colours. Choosing new accents based on the predicted colours for the season, a piece of clothing I am drawn to or a look I have seen on someone is part of the fun of capsule wardrobes for me.

Your core colour will most likely be one of the following neutrals but may change shade or even colour with the seasons; darker in winter and lighter in summer. The items in your core colour will make up a large part of your wardrobe and budget.

Some basic core colours include:

- Navy
- Black
- Grey (from light smoke to dark charcoal)
- Denim
- Cream (from ivory to beige)
- Olive/Khaki
- White
- Camel/taupe/nude

How To Work Out What Clothes You Want In Your Capsule Wardrobe?

There are several ways to decide what clothes are needed in your capsule and different ways work for different people;

Photos: take a photo of every item in your wardrobe and have them printed. You can now easily lay out all your photos and move them around, looking at how items work with each other and putting together different outfits. It is easier to 'see' the full outfit as photos on the table before putting it together with the clothes.

List: listing your favourite items is also an option. Start with a pair of pants and add some tops and then a jacket. Do this with a skirt or another pair of pants. Use your core colour/s and build up outfits using your neutrals and colour accents.

Grid: creating a 4 x 4 or a 4 x 5 square grid allows you to place items and see how many of each you have. Working out how much is enough or how much is too much is a lot easier to do with a grid as you fill in the spaces. This idea is from *The Vivienne Files,* a fantastic blog/website that is well worth a read for Janice's incredible collection of ideas for capsule wardrobe building. *See references for examples and website links*

Claire says: I am mathematically minded and like charts and lists. I prefer to plan my wardrobe using a grid as this allows me to see how many of what item I am selecting and how they work together. Importantly, when the grid is full, I feel a sense of completion and don't look for 'that one piece I think will make everything perfect', because in my mind my wardrobe is complete because the grid is full.

Ellen says: I like to have my own capsule wardrobe guidelines because then I have parameters to work within, but they are not rules I must stick to 100%. My aim is to keep each capsule less than 12 pieces; usually made up for three bottoms, usually jeans, six tops and three toppers. I don't include shoes or accessories in my guidelines, but I keep these at a minimum anyway. I like to write a list each season.

How Many Items Do You Need?

The number of items you have in your capsule wardrobe will depend on your life style, the number of days you wear your clothes and your washing cycle, but it will probably be less than you think.

There are no rules and we are not going to tell you how many items you must have in YOUR capsule wardrobe.

The best way to start is to pick the number you think you need for your first capsule wardrobe and then at the end of the season you can evaluate it. Remember this is an experiment not a test, so you are not trapped by your decision.

We might make it look easy to have a smaller wardrobe but when we started we had many more pieces in our wardrobes than we needed, and we have been able to decrease the size of our wardrobes each season.

It is from continually re-evaluating our wardrobes that we have been able to see how many pieces we REALLY need for our lifestyle.

The Outfit Formula.

Have you ever considered how many different outfit combinations you can make from a certain number of clothing items?

Consider this; you have two pairs of pants, or a pair of pants and a skirt. You have four tops/blouses/t-shirts that work with each of the bottoms. You also have two toppers; either cardigans, jumpers or vests, again that work with all tops and bottoms. So how many outfit combinations can you make?

2 bottoms x 4 tops x 2 toppers = 16 combinations

If you add two different pairs of shoes; flats and boots maybe and even two scarves that work with everything then the maths looks like this;

2 bottoms x 4 tops x 2 toppers x 2 shoes x 2 scarves = 64 different combinations.

So, from those few items you can dress for two months and not wear the same outfit twice. Yes, some of the variations are minimal, but the point is fewer clothes can work for you if they work well together.

This particular idea works well when you have a limit, like travelling. Again, this idea is explained further and illustrated in *The Vivienne Files.*

Here are some ideas you might like to consider while selecting pieces for your capsule wardrobe.

Core or Basic Items

All capsule wardrobe books and websites talk about your core items or your basics. These are the items that will be the base or the blank canvas of your wardrobe, the items that you reach for every day, such as your jeans, pants, black or grey jumper. These are the items that you first think of when putting your daily outfit together.

Claire says: My core items tend to be navy pants and jeans, and plain long sleeve tee shirts and then I add another top in my accent colours. The accent colours vary a little depending on the season, but my core and neutral are the same. Navy is my core colour and cream is my neutral colour. Sometimes a few items in emerald green make an appearance and while they look great with the navy, I can't wear them with the other accent colours. While this isn't quite the 'perfect' coordinating wardrobe, I love emerald green, and feel happy when I wear it – so I do.

Ellen says: My core colours are black, denim and grey year-round and my accent colours change each season. I have just packed away my winter clothing and my accent for winter was blue in several shades. Moving into spring I have accents of coral and khaki. For spring my 12-piece wardrobe consists of 7 core items, with my accents being the other 5 pieces. Some capsules have more core pieces and some less.

Prints and patterns versus plain

A print or patterned item of clothing might be more useful than you think. If you are fortunate enough to find a piece that includes your core colour/s, your neutrals and/or your accent colour/s this item becomes a useful piece in your wardrobe, bringing together different pieces and giving you plenty of options to wear it.

The patterns on a top often give an outfit enough 'interest' so that it may remove the need for accessories like scarves and jewellery. If you prefer an uncluttered look and have stayed away from patterns, try one and see how you feel.

Dressing for your shape and size

Dress for the 'you right now', even if it's not the you, you want to be. Remember the real you and the fantasy you from earlier! There are lots of blogs and websites that provide detailed information on dressing for your body type, how to disguise some features and how to highlight other features.

Statement piece versus work horse piece

A work horse piece is usually a core item that is probably plain, simple and good quality in a neutral colour that can be worn with many different pieces in many ways. A black or navy blazer is an example of a workhorse piece.

A statement piece, much like a statement necklace, may not be worn every day, but is the sort of item worn with the basic core items as the background and gives your outfit a lift, accentuating or identifying your personal style. Your statement piece is likely to change with the seasons or fashion trends. A top with sequins or a bold print is a statement piece.

Transitional capsule

Some seasons are harder to dress for than others. Winter is cold, summer is hot, but spring and autumn can be a mix of both as they lead into and out of the other season. A transitional capsule allows you to transition, or move between two different seasons, usually with more layering items to deal with the colder days and a few short sleeve items for the warmer days.

Chapter 3 Summary

A transitional capsule has more variety but takes more work to put it together as you need to cover seasonal variation

There are numerous ways to plan your capsule wardrobe; take phots, write lists, use a grid. (See reference section)

The number of items in your capsule wardrobe will be the right number for your lifestyle

Use the outfit formula to determine the number of outfit combinations you can make from your clothes.

(a)bottoms x (b)tops x (c)toppers x (d)shoes x (e)scarves = the number of different outfits you can create.

Plan your core items first; their colour and style, and then build on them.

Chapter 3 Activities

The weather where you live determines the size of your season's capsule. What will be your bigger and smaller capsules?_____

_____

Try using the various planning tools. Which one feels best suited to you, your style and personality?

_____

_____

How many pieces do you think you will need in your own capsule wardrobe?

Pants   Skirts   Tops

Toppers   Scarves   Shoes

Jewellery/Other.

My core colour/is/are?_____

My neutral colour is?_____

My accent colours are?_____

Chapter 4

Looking At Your First Capsule

Whatever method you have used to determine your capsule for this season, it is time to and see how it all looks together. If you can, put out everything you have selected, either on the bed or hang them on a rail, a clothes horse or drying rack.

Take a good hard look and ask yourself these questions;

Clothes
Too many? Not enough?

Are there enough pieces to last between wash days?

Does each item function well with my life style?

Do the items work well together?

In a small wardrobe, there is not a lot of room for that piece that only works with one other item.

How does it make me feel?
Having clothes that make you feel great are important when you have a small wardrobe.

Do you have enough core and basic items?
Even though they may initially seem boring, these are the pieces you will turn to every day.

Do you have enough accent items?
These are the items that reflect your personality and will make your wardrobe yours.

Accessories

Scarves

These are the items that will take your outfit from ho-hum to 'wow'. A few scarves that contain some, or if you're lucky, all your core and accent colours, can be used in a variety of ways to finish an outfit of neutral core items.

Simple outfits can look amazing with a scarf, and so to, the same outfit can look quite different when a different scarf is worn.

There are hundreds of YouTube videos showing how to tie and wear scarves of different sizes and shapes. Pick a couple of styles that you like and practice them.

Jewellery

This idea also works with jewellery. An amazing necklace, earrings or a beautiful bracelet can change the look and the focus of an outfit. This collection can be as big or as small as your love for jewellery. While it is practical to also have a capsule wardrobe of jewellery, pieces that are loved and worn can lift a simple outfit to stunning.

Shoes

Comfortable, well-made shoes are an investment and should be part of your clothing budget. Nothing spoils a fabulous outfit faster than a pair of dirty, worn shoes. A few pairs of shoes that work with your core colour (black, navy or tan) are all you really need. However, a statement pair or three are always fun.

Anything missing?

- you've shopped from your own wardrobe
- used the clothes that you love
- applied your chosen method to determine your capsule wardrobe
- checked to see that the items work together
- selected a range of accessories that compliment your choices.

Now it's time to see if there are gaps, what's missing and decide how to fill those gaps.

If you can see, when all your clothes are laid out, that, for example, a plain white t-shirt, or a black blouse or a pair of grey jeans would make all the difference to your wardrobe, increase the number of outfit options you have and really make the whole selection work together, then now is the time to go shopping.

However, if you feel your wardrobe is complete, that it is totally wearable as it is, with sufficient options and combinations to produce outfits that you love, then you don't *need* to go shopping.

It's always interesting to take a walk past your favourite clothing stores to see what in, look at ways of styling what you have or, if something is not working and needs to be replaced.

Make A Wish List And Consider Your Budget

If you've decided you need to go shopping, write a list. It doesn't have to be detailed but if you need a white blouse then don't go thinking about a pink one.

Write a guideline to keep you on track so you can focus on the right item for your new capsule wardrobe.

Look at your clothing budget. If you are at the starting point then it's likely that you will have no money to spend right now and this is where you decide if you really need anything now and if so, how much you can afford to spend?

Claire says: I shop at mid-priced women's wear shops. This suits my budget and it always seems like someone has a sale. I have an amount of money I put away every fortnight and my budget doesn't allow me to buy boutique and designer wear, so I don't look in those stores. Now that I have been doing this for a while, at the beginning of a season I usually have a lump sum that I am able to use to purchase several items to add some fresh ideas to that season's capsule wardrobe. As my savings increase, I am starting to look at buying less but higher quality, and therefore higher priced, core items.

Ellen says: I like shopping for my wardrobe online; I enjoy buying pieces that are not found at every shopping centre so buy from boutiques and from overseas. Over time I have found my favourite brands which have good quality at the right price and these are my go-to stores when I am shopping. I set a seasonal budget, if I don't need much this season I roll the money into the next season. This system allows me to buy fewer pieces which are higher priced, rather than having a wardrobe stuffed with fast fashion. I like to have some money left in my kitty so that I can buy things throughout the season, if I buy everything up front I feel too restricted. I buy most of my clothes (especially core items) at the start of the season and allow myself some wriggle room in case I see something I love as the season goes on.

Chapter 4 Summary

Now that you've created your first capsule, stand back and look.

Enough? Do your clothes look good together?

Are there enough core items to build different outfits?

Are there enough accent items to provide variety and individuality?

Choose accessories to compliment the clothes you have chosen. Shoes, scarves, bags and jewellery make the outfits your own and show your individual style.

Are there are any items of clothing that are missing, that if added to your capsule wardrobe would make a difference to the look and functionality of your wardrobe.

Chapter 4 Activities

How do you feel about your first capsule wardrobe?

_____

_____

Are there enough items to make it work?

_____

_____

Is there anything missing?

_____

_____

Create a shopping list; detailing exactly what the item is that you need. For example; a short sleeved, grey tee shirt, form fitting (sporty/fun), a long sleeved, soft fabric white blouse (relaxed/romantic)

_____

_____

Do you need any accessories?

_____

_____

Chapter 5

Assessing and Making Changes

This next step might just be the most important step in the whole capsule wardrobe process, yet you rarely see it mentioned in blogs and books. According to most pieces we read, once you have arranged your wardrobe with the '10 Essentials' or 'the Capsule Wardrobe must-haves' that's it, it seems, you're done.

But we found over time that we were nowhere near done, it fact we weren't even nearly there. We highly recommend that you sit down at the end of the season and make some notes about what has worked and what hasn't worked in this season's capsule.

Most capsule wardrobe advice focuses on creating a new capsule but the learning and growth that comes from evaluating the capsule at the end of the season is where you gained the most.

Question Your Wardrobe Choices.

At the end of each season, as you pack your clothes away, ask yourself these questions:

- Did I wear it?
- How often did I wear it?
- How did I feel when wearing it?
- Did it go with several other pieces to make multiple outfits?
- Did it suit this season's weather?
- Did it suit my lifestyle?
- Which accessories worked with the piece?

The Ten Things I Learnt From My Capsule Wardrobe

When you assess your wardrobe, if you can, write a list of ten things you have learnt from this season's capsule. Be as honest and specific as you can be. Write about what worked for the stage of life you are in now and what made you feel like your best self and what did not.

Why ten? We found the first five are almost always easy and somewhat obvious, but it was around number seven that we had our *ah-ha* moment. If you can write more than ten, do so, but it's when you must stop and think that reality dawns.

Use your answers to help build your next season's capsule and then tuck the list into your clothes as you pack them away at the end of this season. Next year when you pull out these pieces again, you will be reminded of what worked and what didn't, and you can build on this knowledge as you create that season's capsule again.

Ellen says: I wrote my list of 10 things in two parts, things I learnt and things I know. Things I learnt were new information I had learnt about me from the capsule. Things I know were things I had confirmed worked for me this capsule. For example, after my spring capsule I learnt that I need to have lots of cold and hot weather clothes in my spring capsule because the weather is so variable where I live. I confirmed that I prefer wearing pants and my favourite pants to wear are jeans.

Claire says: The first time I seriously created a capsule wardrobe using the process outlined in this book was for a winter season. At the end of the season when I wrote my list of ten, I discovered some interesting things. Even though I thought my clothing selection was right on, I found I had more clothes than I needed and was passing over the heavy weight jumpers on a regular basis for others that were layering favourites. Surprisingly, the pieces I wore the most were patterned tops. I had though I preferred plain block colours that I could add interest with a scarf. Thinking about this, I realised that a pattered top added the same interest that the scarf provided, with one less item to wear. When at work, not having a scarf around my neck just made my outfit more streamlined and less 'fiddly'. I wore the same three pairs of shoes almost all the time. While I love heels, on a day to day basis, I need a low to medium heel.

How Did Your Clothes Stand Up To Wear?

As you pack last season's capsule away, it is also time to assess each garment with a critical eye.

- What state is it in?
- Did it stand up to a season of wear?
- Does it have pilling or holes?
- Is it worn out?
- Is it stretched or misshapen?
- Is the colour fading?

If any of these are the case and this piece was one you loved and got a lot of wear from, then you may want to replace it next year. Make a note so that you know what to look for when shopping for that season's next capsule wardrobe.

We don't suggest throwing away or donating any pieces from your wardrobe at this stage. Sometimes clothes can look stale after a season of wear but next year when you unpack, it will feel fresh and new again and you will enjoy wearing it for another season.

Any pieces that have seen better days and need replacing are best kept until next year, so you can use it as a template when shopping. If you get rid of it now all you will have is a note to add a "grey top" to your wish list, when what you really loved about this piece is it was a ¾ raglan sleeve top with a high low hemline made of a cotton/spandex blend. There is a big difference!

Assess Your Accessories

This is also the time to go through an analysis process with your jewellery, scarves, shoes and hand bags. It can be too easy to keep items in the accessories category that never get used because they are often smaller and stored outside the main wardrobe.

When analysing this category, you may find yourself noting the pieses you need as much those you don't.

Would a scarf made up of your accent colours have helped tie your wardrobe together?

Are your children getting older, so a smaller handbag would work better for your needs now?

Remember the more time and effort you put into this analysis step the better your subsequent capsule wardrobes will be. A thorough evaluation will save you time and money in the long run and will help you curate a capsule that makes you feel your best every day.

It becomes easier each time you select your new season's capsule wardrobe as you learn more about yourself and your style. However, there is no definitive answer to any of the questions we ask. Your wardrobe is a moving and changing creation and it reflects the moves and changes in your life.

Ellen says: Go through this process every time you change out your capsule and you will be amazed at how much you can learn about yourself! Each time you do it you will fine tune your capsule and make it more cohesive and better suited to your life.

Claire says: By considering your accessories at the same time as assessing your past capsule and selecting your next one, you are extending the options of a smaller wardrobe and creating your signature style.

Chapter 5 Summary

Reflection and assessment are important steps in creating your capsule wardrobe.

The assessment at the end of a season is an important exercise in learning and growth, in both creating your capsule and understanding your style.

Question your choices; choices in clothes, accessories, style and taste.

At the end of a season write a list of 10 observations, if you can, that you have learnt about your style and your capsule wardrobe selection. Include thoughts on what worked and what didn't.

Chapter 5 Activities

Write a list of at least 10 observations you've made this season; about your style and your capsule wardrobe.

_____

_____

_____

_____

Did you have the right accessorise?

_____

_____

Too many or not enough?

_____

_____

Did your clothes stand up to regular wear?

- What brands performed well?
- What brands underperformed?

_____

_____

Chapter 6

The Next Capsule

Now is the time to take what you have learned from the self-assessment of your last capsule and create your next one.

Remember, if it is spring or autumn, a transitional season capsule requires a little more thought as it blends two seasons. It is either still warm but will get cooler or still cool but will be getting warmer. Whatever you choose, allow for warmer days with cooler morning and evenings.

Claire says: as I write this I have just changed from my winter to spring capsule wardrobe. However, the weather has taken a turn and it may as well still be winter. My current wardrobe consists of layers, pieces that can be taken off during the day if it warms up and layered in the mornings and evenings when it is cooler. There are two heavier weight pieces; woollen jumpers that are being worn now and two short sleeve tops for the warmer end of the season. The remaining items are long sleeve tops that can be layered with cardigans and jackets.

Ellen says: My transition capsules, spring and autumn, need to be bigger than my winter and summer ones because there is so much variation. These are also traditionally longer seasons where I live – so I can't always follow the dates for my capsules. You might find the same where you live, or you might have a short spring followed by a long hot summer, so your summer wardrobe needs to start early. Making your capsule unique to where you live is much more important than following the dates on the calendar.

Selecting the Next Capsule

Use your preferred selection method to pick the right number of clothes for the upcoming season; a list, numbers, photos, grid or formula.

Follow the same principles as when you selected your first capsule wardrobe;

- consider your lifestyle – travel, meetings, formal occasions, Stay at Home Mum, part time work.
- do the items work together? – look at photos, lay the clothes on your bed, hang them on an airer or rail.
- apply all the things you have learnt from your analysis of your first capsule wardrobe.
- now choose your accessories; scarves, shoes, bags and jewellery to get the maximum wear from each item.

Here is a reminder of the process as well as some tips for packing away last season's clothes.

Change Over Day

- empty your wardrobe and place your clothes on the bed or on a rail
- vacuum out your wardrobe getting rid of any dust and cobwebs
- unpack next season's selection and hang them in the wardrobe.
- if they need ironing or steaming do it as you go. Set up the ironing board or steamer near your wardrobe, play some of your favourite music or listen to a podcast as you work
- get our scarves, jewellery, bags and shoes that you have chosen to be part of this season's capsule.
- once everything is in the wardrobe – admire it.
- pack away or store all the clothes that are clean.
- wash any woollens or items that need it. Air and brush down jackets and coats
- blazers and winter coats benefit from a professional clean and press. Take them to the dry cleaners if you can.
- check over your shoes. Discard any that are truly worn out and irreparable.

- any that are well worn can be reheeled and resoled by a cobbler or shoe repair shop. This will give you another season's wear from your favourite shoes.
- wipe over all synthetic shoes, use a clean shoe brush to brush up suede shoes and use some polish and elbow grease to give leather shoes a good clean. Packed away clean and repaired they are ready for next season.
- pack away scarves, jewellery and bags you know you won't need this coming season.
- remember to add the notes you made as a reminder for next time.

Chapter 6 Summary

When planning your next capsule, consider the weather now, and as you move through the coming season.

Repeat your preferred method to select your next capsule. Follow the same process as the first time, using what you've learnt after your assessment.

Follow the changeover day procedure, giving your physical wardrobe a spring clean and enjoying the process of packing away last seasons clothes and unpacking this season's clothes.

Pack away off-season accessories with off season clothes.

Don't forget to add in any notes or information you've written to help put together this capsule next time.

Chapter 6 Activities

What is the weather going to be like during this season you are preparing for?

_____

_____

Are there any special items of clothing you will need? E.g.: swimsuit, snow boots.

_____

_____

_____

What is your preferred method for selecting this season's capsule? What items will you include?

_____

_____

_____

Remember to make some notes to keep with the clothes you re packing away. Include outfits you liked, clothes that you would like to replace, items that you might need to buy and your list of 10 observations.

Chapter 7

Other Capsules

It's all well and good having a great capsule wardrobe for your work or everyday clothes, but what about the rest of your wardrobe? What about your underwear, loungewear, active wear, formal outfits, sleepwear and travel wear?

You can create any size capsule wardrobe for each of these categories. Just keep in mind that the size of the capsule needs to represent the importance of that event in your life. Remember - no dressing the 'fantasy you'.

Underwear

This will be an individual requirement for everyone but let's be practical. Do you really need more than 3 or 4 everyday bras and a couple of 'special' ones?

Make sure you have exactly what you need for your wardrobe. If you wear strapless dresses, then a strapless bra is essential, if you never wear dresses that might show your bra strap then you don't really need a strapless bra.

Wear the correct size and shaped underwear for you and your outfit. Try and have a look from behind to make sure all is as you imagine it to be.

Be brave and have your bra professionally fitted. Buy from a specialist shop or department store, preferable not off the rack in a chain store.

Believe it when you hear that quality undergarments make all the difference in your outer appearance. No matter the name or cost of your top or dress, a badly fitting bra will spoil the look, so have it professionally fitted and replace it when the elastic starts to look stretched and tatty.

Think about the colours you buy and how they will look under the clothes you have chosen.

Do you need to wear matching underwear sets? Of course you don't, but it will make you feel nice and a beige bra and beige knickers is still a matching set.

Underwear need not be expensive wisps of lace, unless that is your garment of choice. Just make sure it fits and can't be seen.

Remember to consider your undergarments every time you change over your capsule wardrobe.

Sleepwear

This is an outfit where many of us don't pay a lot of attention. 'I'm in bed, no one will see me,' 'I want to be comfortable, it doesn't matter.' But it does matter; to you, to how you feel and what you are saying to and about yourself.

Throw out the holey yoga or track pants and the old t-shirts and buy yourself some sleepwear. It can be as simple or as luxurious as you'd like, but it just needs to be presentable sleepwear that makes you feel good.

We suggest two sets of summer sleepwear and two sets of winter sleepwear; one to wear and one in the wash. If you need something for trans-seasonal months, then find something that suits your needs. You can choose a nightie, nightshirt, short pjs or long pjs depending on your climate and sleeping habits. If you prefer to sleep nude, then that's a whole capsule you have saved yourself, but maybe you can indulge in a luxurious gown.

And while you are looking at sleepwear, maybe consider a matching gown. You will probably need one so why not get one that works with your sleepwear, either part of a set or a matching or contrasting colour. This will help you feel 'put together' without taking much effort and not everyone has the energy to make an effort first thing in the morning.

Loungewear

Lounge wear is what you change into when you get home or when you want to change out of 'work' or 'good' clothes. Loungewear may be your 'comfy' clothes, but they are not your slobby clothes.

Loungewear is not an excuse to wear old, tatty, holey clothes that once belonged to someone else or favourites you've had for years that you can't part with. Your partner's stained tracksuit pants with a hole in the knee and an old faded jumper are not doing you any favours.

Make sure you have enough for your needs, that they are soft and comfortable, but fit nicely and look nice together. Try a pair of soft black or navy pants and a nice fitting, colour coordinating top or soft and snugly jumper. You don't need a large collection, just enough to suit your needs.

Travel

This is one of our favourite capsules and one that can be fun to put together. There are lots of websites that talk about travel capsules and offer all sorts of advice and formulas to create exactly what you need. There are some links and further information in the resources section of this book.

With a small capsule wardrobe, you can easily take everything you'll need even if you are away for a few weeks. Depending on where you are going, try to dress as you would every day at home. While this may not work on a beach or skiing holiday, it probably will on a typical tourist holiday or family visit.

As with our transitional capsules, where weather conditions vary, layering is always a safe option. Remember to add some scarves or jewellery as they can change up the look and feel of an outfit without adding bulk and weight to your case.

Active Wear

If you need a selection of work out gear, try and buy it together. You don't have to spend a fortune on designer pieces, but tops and bottoms that work well together will make you feel confident and put together before you hit the gym.

Decide how many sets you need, based on the number of days you need to wear sportswear and the number of times you wash per week. A drawer full is not necessary if you need two outfits a week, but forever looking for something to wear when you work out daily is just frustrating.

Replace pieces when they become saggy or start to look tired and worn and check your look from behind. Is the material thick enough to cover what needs to be covered?

Sportswear and gym clothes are just that. Try not to get into the habit of wearing sport wear as every day clothes. You have a capsule wardrobe of clothes you love, enjoy wearing those and keep the sportswear for the gym.

Remember - yoga pant are not everyday pants!

Formal Wear

We all get invited to weddings, work functions, special dinners and, unfortunately, funerals. Having a small formal wardrobe can have you looking stylish at any event without the last-minute shopping panic – and the associated overspending! A pair of black pants or a skirt, two or three appropriate tops and a jacket will suit almost any occasions. If you prefer a dress, then two or three dresses in different colours and styles would be useful.

Have a jacket, pair of shoes and a small handbag/clutch that goes with everything. If you find yourself in formal occasions multiple times a week, then this is another capsule that you can create, applying all the rules from the earlier chapters.

Chapter 7 Summary

Thinking of your other clothes as capsules, allows you to curate them in a logical way.

Other capsules can include;

- Sleepwear
- Active or sportswear
- Formal wear
- Underwear
- Loungewear

Follow the same rules when putting together these smaller capsules.

Make sure these capsules cover your needs.

Chapter 7 Activities

How many additional capsules can you see in
your wardrobe?

_____

_____

Which ones need some work?

_____

_____

How many items do you need in each of these
capsules?

_____

_____

Chapter 8

Final Thoughts

Once you have completed a few wardrobe reviews, you will have learnt a lot about your wardrobe, about yourself and your individual style. Having a well curated wardrobe requires introspection and reveals your true self in your sense of style.

We have found the most important part of any capsule wardrobe we create is the assessment at the end of the season. Making notes and asking ourselves questions helps establish and refine our style.

It is important to remember;

- Being able to say goodbye to your fantasy self and loving the life you live now, is one of the many benefits that come from the process of refining your style and then your wardrobe.

- You will be able to save money, now and in the future. No longer buying pieces that don't work, no more wardrobe orphans, no more buying pieces that don't feel right, just because you read you should own it this season.

- Getting dressed will be so much easier. No more, 'what should I wear?' that once plagued your mornings. Once you are dressed you won't think about your outfit again for the rest of the day – a small luxury that can feel quite life changing.

- You will find yourself a much more confident shopper who feels sure in her choices, and your wardrobe will reflect this new found inner confidence.

We hope you have found this book useful and that you enjoy the journey you are on; learning about yourself and your sense of style. Enjoy the process and have fun with your clothes.

Remember, when your favourite blog tells you what every woman must have in her wardrobe this season, use those ideas as a guide; change the colour, the style and the fabric to suit you and your lifestyle.

There is no right or wrong way to create a capsule wardrobe Each time you curate and plan your next season's wardrobe you will learn from your past wardrobes and you will always get better at defining your very own curated capsule wardrobe.

Resources

Here are some of the blogs that we enjoy and that have inspired us to create our capsule wardrobes.

The Vivienne Files

www.theviviennefiles.com

The Daily Connoisseur

www.dailyconnoisseur.blogspot.com

How To Be Chic

www.howtobechic.com

Un-fancy

www.un-fancy.com

Project 333

www.bemorewithless.com/project-333

The Travel Medley

www.thetravelmedley.com/author/thetravelmedley

The Anna Edit

www.theannaedit.com

Shot From The Street

www.shotfromthestreet.com

Styling You

www.stylingyou.com.au

Wardrobe Oxygen

www.wardrobeoxygen.com

Wardrobe Planning Grid.

This grid is similar to the one you will find on The Vivienne Files (www.theviviennefiles.com) and the initial idea came from that blog and has been adapted for personal use. There is a lot of information about the '4x4 Wardrobe' on The Vivienne Files and some great examples showing how effective it is selecting a capsule wardrobe.

Four items of clothing in your core colour				
Four items in your neutral or another core colour				
Four tops that go with both colours				
Four items that round out your wardrobe, a dress, a pair of jeans etc				

How to Sell Clothes and Accessories On-line

Decide if the item is truly worth the time and hassle of selling online. Chanel purse gets a tick; slightly stretched knit from Target store gets a cross. Items not worth selling can be donated (if in good condition), given to a friend or if there are any rips, holes etc. then the item needs to go in the bin.

Decide how to sell the item. There are websites dedicated to selling second hand high end luxury brands, there is eBay, Gumtree and also Facebook groups for locals and particular brands. This step can take a little research (try searching for the item on each of the sites listed below) but can make a difference in the price and speed of the sale.

Again consider if the item is worth selling. While searching eBay you can look at the sold history and see what pieces similar to yours went for. If there is a lot of examples of similar items selling for $2.99 maybe it would be better to give the item away?

Photo Time. Take lots of photos of the item in the best natural light you can find. This will probably be in the mid-morning and if in

Australia, near a north facing window. Natural light always makes for better photos! Make sure you take photos from different angles, close ups of any important features (such as the label and size, detailing, lace, buttons and logos etc) and also take photos of any faults in the garment. Make sure you get a photo which has a good likeness of the actual colour of the fabric - shadows or bright lights can alter the way the colour shows up in the photo.

Measure the garment, most people do this lying flat and note down as much detail as you can. Google becomes your friend to look up exact style names and more info on the type of fabrics used. The more detail you can give the more chance you have of selling an item for a good price. Have a look at the listings for new items from your favourite online store and try to match that level of detail. It might include washing instructions – "This knit is hand wash only, I have always followed the care label and dried flat in the shade" or even a style guide – "I loved wearing this top with jeans and neutral flats for a summer day out". You need to be a salesperson here!

Decide on a realistic, achievable price. You want the item to sell so be pragmatic. Sitting in your wardrobe it was worth $0, not the $100 you paid for it ten years ago. Would you rather have $20 in your hand tomorrow or have the jacket still hanging in your wardrobe six months from now because you overpriced it? eBay is helpful here because you can set a low starting price (which helps attract customers) and in the end the final price will be a realistic indication of the market.

Get online, go to your chosen platform and start listing. Different platforms and even different categories within platforms have different rules on selling so I can't tell you exactly what this step will look like for you. You can google "How to list an item on..." to find a current up to date step by step walkthrough. Just remember that the more detail you can offer a buyer the more secure they will feel buying your item. Always put up as many photos as the platform allows.

Answer questions as they come in and keep an eye on your item - if it hasn't sold within a week (or the timeframe chosen for your auction on eBay) then it's time to stop and think. Is it overpriced? Is there any important information I missed giving the buyer? Are the photos good enough? Should I try a different platform?

Always set yourself a timeframe - we don't want you having a bag of clothes sitting in your wardrobe for a year waiting to sell. Maybe after two weeks without selling the items could be donated instead?

If the item sells then package it carefully and send to the buyer only once payment has been made. Postage costs can vary so have an idea of how much the item will cost to send before listing it for sale. Australia Post has prepaid satchels in different weight sizes which can be posted anywhere in Australia. If you have a few items to sell you could buy a pack of prepaid satchels and have them ready to go at home.

Find something fun to do with the money you made! Put it in your wardrobe budget or shout a girlfriend to dinner out. Celebrate! Don't think about how much the item cost you and how little it sold for, that's a futile exercise. Be happy that your item has gone to someone who will love and wear it and you have money that you didn't have while it was sitting unworn in your wardrobe.

Here are some **online platforms** for selling clothes and accessories:

www.therealreal.com For high end and luxury brands

www.ebay.com The popular auction site has lots of potential buyers but also has lots of competition so might not give you the highest prices. eBay is a great place to do an initial search for price comparison.

www.gumtree.com less fees than eBay but not as large an audience. In Australia there are not a lot of clothes on Gumtree but it might be different where you live.

Facebook buy/swap/sell groups. Facebook groups are free and are a great way to find local buyers who can pay cash on pick up. There are specific groups for kids clothing, maternity clothing, plus sized clothing and groups for many specific brands of clothing. When you write up a listing on Facebook you can choose to have the item posted in numerous groups so even more potential buyers see it. Make sure you put a note in your listing that says it is advertised elsewhere (sometimes the acronym LOOP – listed on other places is used). Facebook does not have a payment system like eBay so it is a case of buyer and seller beware; never post an item until you have received payment.